Sahir Omrani
Achraf Sarraj

Cholecystectomy after acute biliary pancreatitis

Sahir Omrani
Achraf Sarraj

Cholecystectomy after acute biliary pancreatitis

indications for intraoperative cholangiography

ScienciaScripts

Imprint

Any brand names and product names mentioned in this book are subject to trademark, brand or patent protection and are trademarks or registered trademarks of their respective holders. The use of brand names, product names, common names, trade names, product descriptions etc. even without a particular marking in this work is in no way to be construed to mean that such names may be regarded as unrestricted in respect of trademark and brand protection legislation and could thus be used by anyone.

Cover image: www.ingimage.com

This book is a translation from the original published under ISBN 978-620-6-72571-8.

Publisher:
Sciencia Scripts
is a trademark of
Dodo Books Indian Ocean Ltd. and OmniScriptum S.R.L publishing group

120 High Road, East Finchley, London, N2 9ED, United Kingdom
Str. Armeneasca 28/1, office 1, Chisinau MD-2012, Republic of Moldova, Europe
Printed at: see last page
ISBN: 978-620-8-20847-9

CHOLECYSTECTOMY AFTER ACUTE BILIARY PANCREATITIS: INDICATIONS FOR INTRAOPERATIVE CHOLANGIOGRAPHY.

CONTENTS

INTRODUCTION

Acute pancreatitis (AP) is a fairly common condition worldwide. It accounts for 4% of abdominal pain syndromes in the United States (1).

There is an 8-10% mortality rate and 30-40% morbidity in severe forms. Lithiasis and alcoholism are the main causes of this disease. (1) In Tunisia, lithiasis is the most common aetiology.

The risk factors for the latter are: female gender, age > 70 years and vesicular lithiasis of less than 5 mm (2).

The pathophysiology of lithiasis is that a vesicular calculus migrates into the main pancreatic duct, creating an increase in intraductal pressure and obstructing the elimination of pancreatic secretions. (3)

Trypsinogen is thus inappropriately activated, leading to pancreatic autodigestion (4)

For this reason, the American Society for Gastrointestinal Endoscopy (ASGE) considers biliary BP to be a predictive sign of lithiasis of the main bile duct (5). (LVBP)

There is much debate about whether and how to investigate this type of lithiasis. Endoscopic ultrasound appears to be the most effective tool for diagnose LVBP. (6)

Endoscopic retrograde cholangiopancreatography (ERCP) is a highly effective diagnostic and, above all, therapeutic method. (7)

Magnetic resonance cholangiopancreatography (MRCP) is the most widely used imaging technique, with results similar to endoscopic ultrasound except for stones less than 5 mm in size (8).

Intraoperative cholangiography (IOC) is the reference intraoperative examination for the diagnosis of BVG lithiasis (9).

In our country, intraoperative cholangiography is still the most commonly used method to search for possible LVBP during cholecystectomy after any biliary PA.

Several studies have shown that vacuity of the main bile duct (MBD) is present in the vast majority of cases. In this study, we therefore propose to review the formal indication for CPO in this condition by looking for factors predictive of the presence of LVBP.

PATIENTS AND METHODS

I. Type and objectives of the study :

We conducted a retrospective study in the visceral surgery department of the CHU Mongi Slim in La Marsa from 1 January 2016 to 31 December 2021. We collected 107 cases. This work made it possible to collect epidemiological, clinical, paraclinical and therapeutic data on this pathology. The aim of our work was to study the factors predictive of the presence of lithiasis of the main biliary tract following acute pancreatitis of biliary origin and thus to review the indication for intraoperative cholangiography in these cases.

II. Inclusion criteria :

All patients who underwent surgery after acute pancreatitis of

who had undergone intraoperative cholangiography.

III. Non-inclusion criteria :

Patients who had a preoperative BILI MRI and/or ERCP.

Patients who have not had CPO for any reason.

IV. Exclusion criteria :

Files that cannot be used.

V. Methodology :

The data was collected from the department's archives.

To study our series and, in particular, to obtain all the parameters for each patient, we drew up data sheets summarising the patients' medical records.

We have specified the following parameters:

■Age

■Sex

■Medical and surgical history

■Functional signs (pain, fever, jaundice)

■Physical signs (fever, jaundice, abdominal examination)

■Biological parameters (blood count, renal function tests, liver function tests, inflammatory response tests)

■Abdominal ultrasound data (LV, dilatation of the

■VBP, dilatation of VBIH, LVBP)

■Abdominal CT scan data (LV, dilated LVP, dilated HVBV, LVBP, stage)

■Intraoperative findings (cholecystitis, cystic duct dilatation)

■CPO findings (dilatation of the VBP: the diameter of the VBP was estimated approximately by comparing it with the diameter of the trocars, dilatation of the VBIH, presence of LVBP, duodenal passage)

■Action based on the results of the CPO.

JUDGING CRITERIA AND DEFINITIONS

I. Diagnosis of acute pancreatitis :

A positive diagnosis of acute pancreatitis is made when two of the following three criteria are present:

• Typical pain.

• An increase in lipasemia above three times normal.

• Imaging showing signs of pancreatitis (CT scan, MRI or ultrasound).

It should be noted that amylasemia testing has been abandoned according to French recommendations and that CT scans are sometimes used for diagnostic purposes in the event of an unlabelled abdominal emergency.

II. Dilatation of the main bile duct :

Several studies have been carried out and several scores have been established for the presence of LVBP. All took into account the dilatation of the BPV on ultrasound. Depending on the study, the reference diameters varied between 6 and 12 mm.

We took the lowest value as the reference value and, for the purposes of our study, considered the BPV to be dilated when its diameter exceeds 6 mm.

III. Severity of pancreatitis :

Three degrees of severity have been established according to the revised classification of the

Atlanta 2012 conference:

•mild BP: no local or systemic complications (systemic complications being defined as aggravation of a pre-existing comorbidity) or visceral failure.

•Moderately severe BP: one or more local or systemic complications, or transient visceral failure.

•Severe AP: persistent visceral failure, which may affect one or more organs.

In our study, we considered pancreatitis that did not meet the criteria for mild acute pancreatitis to be severe.

Abdominal CT scans were performed in all patients. The average delay was 5 days after the onset of symptoms.

IV. Stage of pancreatitis and aetiological assessment :

The stages were established according to Balthazar's classification as follows:

Table 1: Stages of pancreatitis

Stage	Computed tomography data
A	Normal pancreas
B	Focal or diffuse enlargement of the pancreatic gland
C	Densification of peripancreatic fat
D	Single necrotic flow
E	At least two necrotic flows or one containing bubbles air

Abdominal ultrasound was also performed in all patients to look for vesicular lithiasis as an aetiology for pancreatitis. This was done during hospitalisation. It also looked for dilatation of the bile ducts and the presence of any LVBP.

V. Indication for surgery :

Our study concerns acute pancreatitis of biliary origin and all our patients underwent surgery with the aim of performing a cholecystectomy (to eliminate the reservoir) and a CPO (to search for LVBP). The timing of the operation was as follows:

▶ For stages A, B and C pancreatitis: the operation was performed during the same hospital stay (between day 6ième and day 14ième).

▶ For stages D and E pancreatitis: the operation was delayed until after the necrosis had been checked by CT scan.

VI. Cholangiography :

The aim of intraoperative cholangiography was mainly to search for LVBP. It was performed through a transcystic drain (DTC).

The LVBP appears as a lacunar image or a cup-shaped stop in the VBP. On CPO, we also look for dilatation of the PVB and/or the intrahepatic bile ducts (IHBD) as well as good or poor duodenal passage of the contrast medium.

STATISTICAL ANALYSIS

Data was entered using SPSS 26.0 statistical software.

The statistical processing of the data included a descriptive and an analytical component.

I. Descriptive study

Qualitative variables were expressed by their frequencies and proportions. Quantitative variables were expressed in terms of their means, standard deviation and

the range (extreme values).

II. Analytical study

We performed a univariate and multivariate analysis of factors predictive of main bile duct lithiasis.

Two means were compared using Student's t-test.

Frequencies were compared using Pearson's chi-square test when the application conditions were met, and Fisher's test in other cases.

A multivariate analysis was established by calculating a logistic regression.

A relationship between variables is considered to be significant if the correlation coefficient "p" is :: 0,05.

III. Ethical and legal considerations

We had no conflicts of interest in relation to the content of our study.

We respected patients' anonymity. Access to the archives was authorised by the head of the general surgery department at the CHU Mongi Slim in La Marsa.

RESULTS

A. Descriptive study

I. Characteristics of the population studied

1.Age :

The extremes of age at the time of the operation were 18 and 87, with an average of 51.59. The age group most represented in our series was between 33 and 69. years (58.9%).

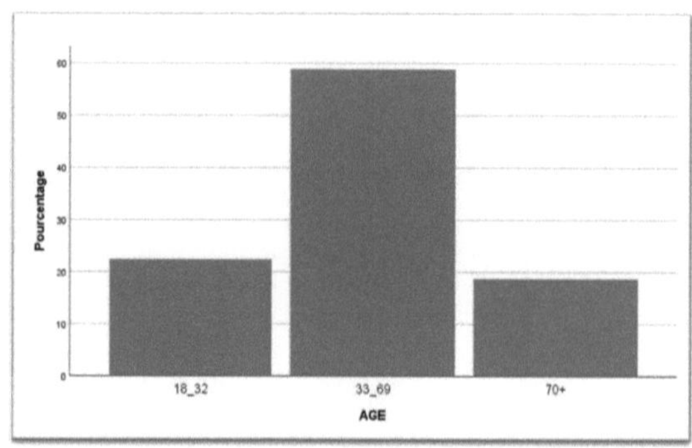

Figure 1: Breakdown of patients by age group

2. Gender :

Our series included 83 women (77.5%) and 24 men (22.5%), giving a sex ratio of 0.28 (Figure 2).

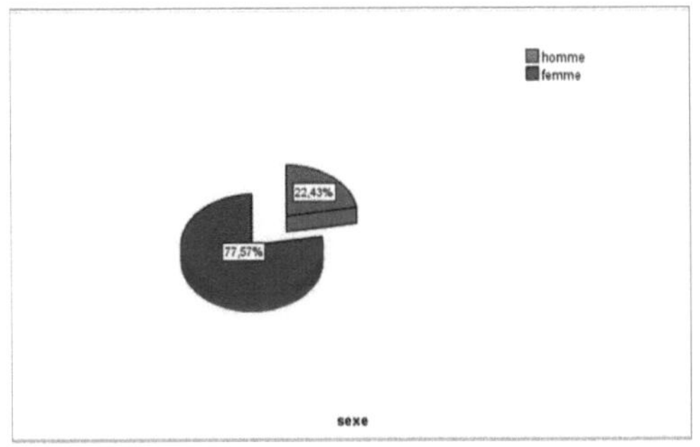

Figure 2: Breakdown of patients by gender

3. ASA score :

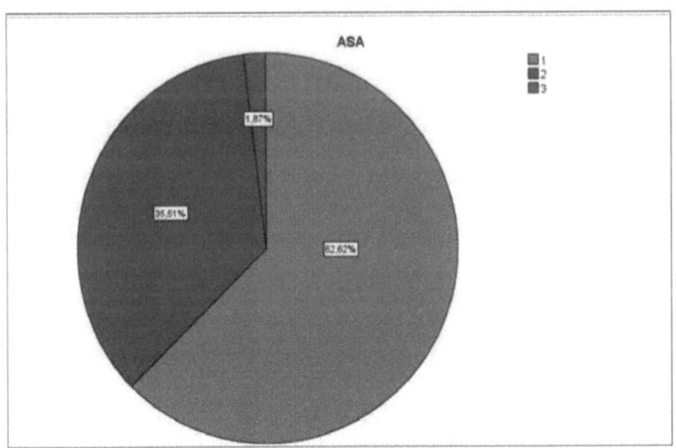

Figure 3: Distribution of patients by ASA score

1.4. Medical history :

Thirty-nine patients (36.5%) had a medical history. Hypertension was the most common medical history (27.1% of patients).

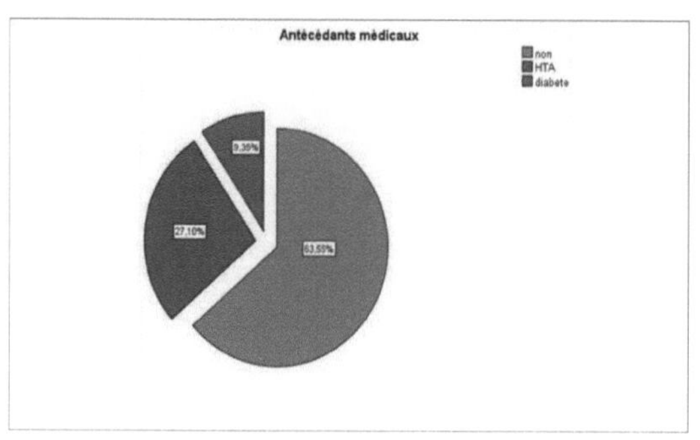

Figure 4: Breakdown of patients by medical history

2. Clinical examination data

Data from the clinical examination on admission were recorded in all the files. Six patients had a temperature above 37.8, and six were icteric. No icteric patient had a fever. Dark urine was found in 2 cases, discoloured stools in only one, and there was no pruritus in all patients. Only one patient had a triad of jaundice, discoloured stools and urine. dark. The vast majority (88%) of patients had none of these clinical signs. Typical hepatic colic was found in 39 patients (36.4%).

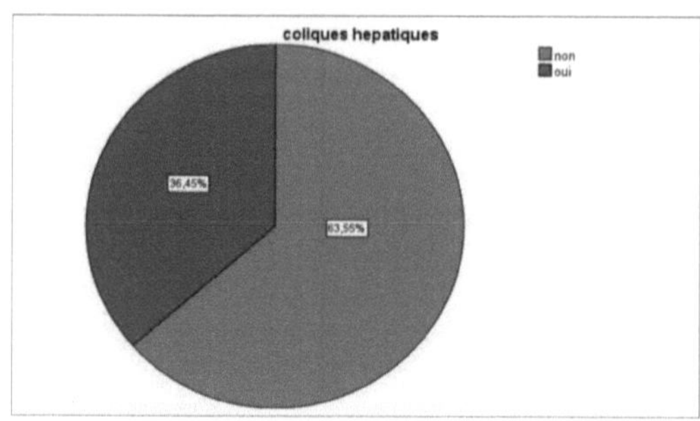

Figure 5: Frequency of hepatic colic

Twenty-two patients (20.56%) had severe pancreatitis.

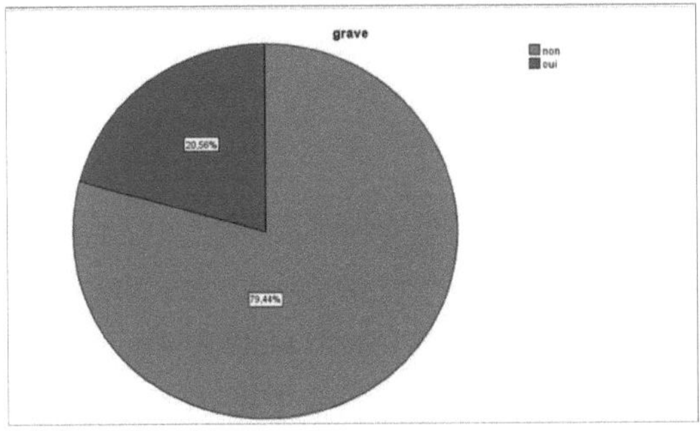

Figure 6: Breakdown by severity of pancreatitis

III. Biological data

1. Total bilirubin levels

Total bilirubin (BT) levels were available for all our patients. The results were as follows:

Table 2: Total bilirubin levels

Average30	.731 mmol/L
Minimum3	.0 mmol/L
Maximum270	.0 mmol/L

2.Conjugated bilirubin levels

In 15 of our patients, the conjugated bilirubin (CB) level was was not available.

Table 3: Conjugated bilirubin levels

Average	15,375
Minimum	0,5
Maximum	150,0

3. Cytolysis

Aspartate aminotransferase (ASAT) and alanine aminotransferase (ALAT) levels were not found in 3 cases. The mean values were 185.6 and 167.6 IU/L respectively.

Table 4: Transaminase levels

	ASAT	ALAT
Average	185,69	167,60
Minimum	12	3
Maximum	1117	840

4.Alkaline phosphatase (ALP) levels was available in only 18 patients. It varied between

9 and 467 IU/L.	Table 5: PAL rates
Average	194,86
Minimum	9
Maximum	467

5. Gamma-glutamyl-transferase (GGT) levels was available in only 22 patients. The results in IU/L are as follows:

Table 6: GGT levels

Average	186,18
Minimum	14
Maximum	450

IV. Imaging data

1. Ultrasound

1.1. Dilatation of the VBP

Abdominal ultrasound data were not found in 3 patients. Of the 104 remaining patients, 27 (25.96%) had a dilated VBP.

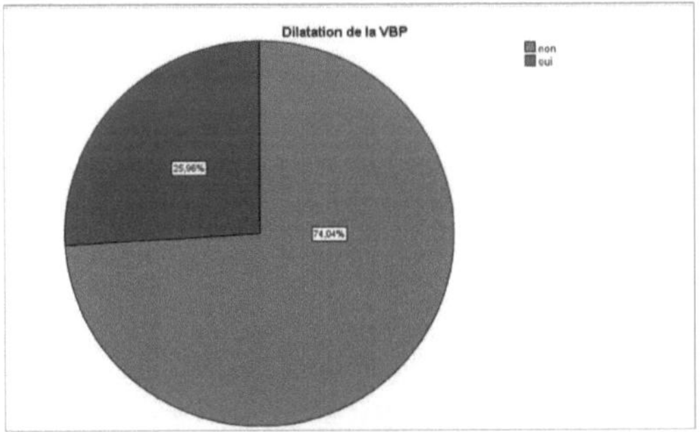

Figure 7: Frequency of dilatation of the BPV on ultrasound scan

1.2. Dilatation of VBIH

Dilatation of the VBIH was observed in 14 of the 104 cases analysed, i.e. 13.1%.

17

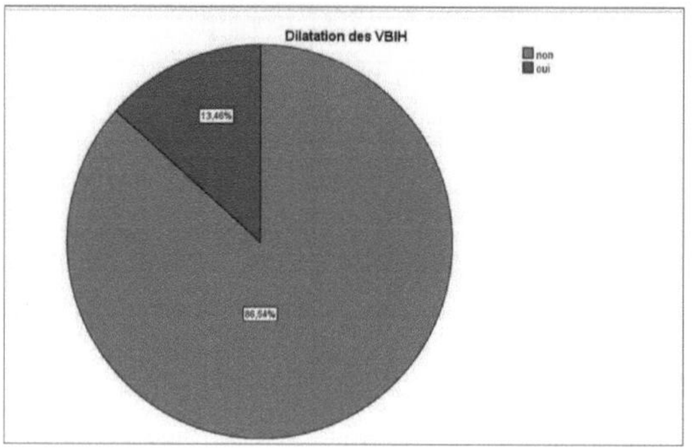

Figure 8: Frequency of HBV dilatation on ultrasonography

1.3. LVBP

Twelve of the 104 patients who underwent ultrasound had LVBP, i.e. 11.2%.

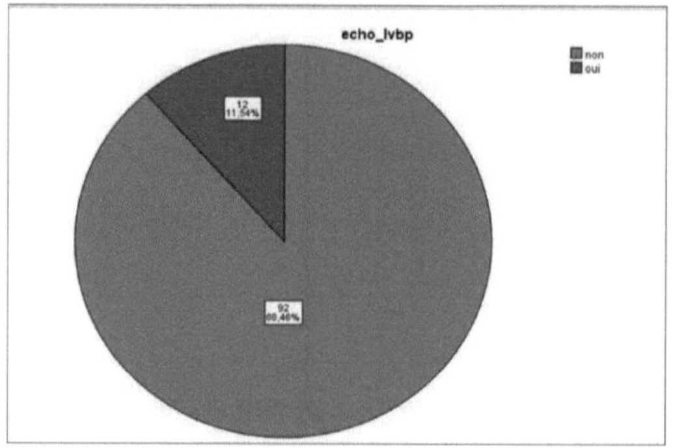

Figure 9: LVBP rate at ultrasound scan

2. Computed tomography

All our patients underwent a staging CT scan. The results were as follows:

2.1. Dilatation of the VBP

Of the 107 patients, 28 had a dilated VBP (26.4%).

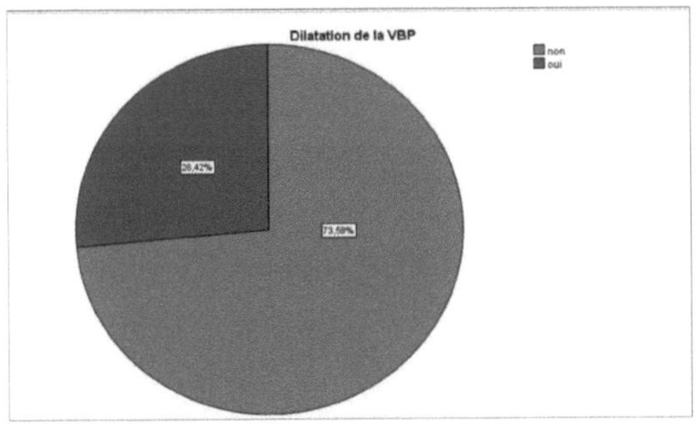

Figure 10: Frequency of dilatation of the VBP on CT scan

2.2. Dilatation of VBIH

Dilatation of the VBIH was observed in 15 of the 107 cases analysed, i.e. 14%.

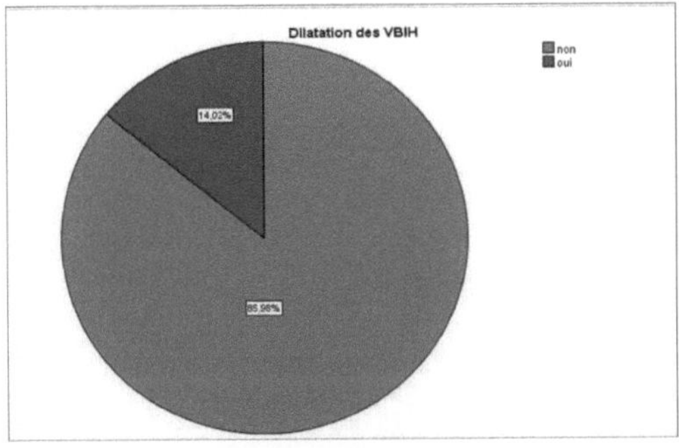

Figure 11: Frequency of dilatation of the VBIH on CT scan

2.3. LVBP

LVBP was present on CT in 8 patients (7.5%).

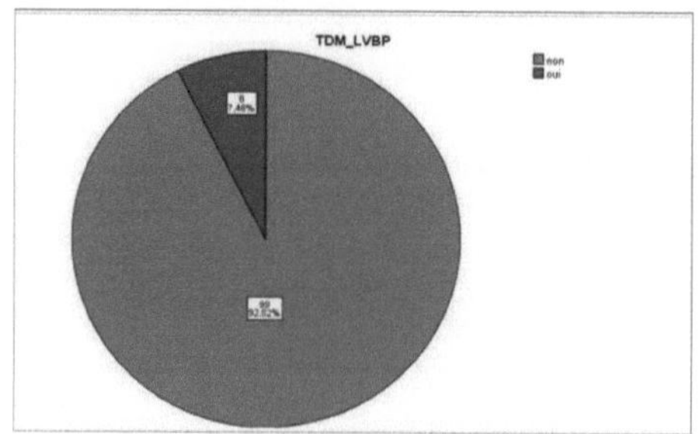

Figure 12: LVBP rate on CT scan

2.4. Stage of pancreatitis

The distribution of patients according to the stage of pancreatitis was as follows:

- 13 for stage A, i.e. 12.15

- 39 for stage B, i.e. 36.45%.

- 32 for stage C, i.e. 29.91%.

- 6 for stage D, i.e. 5.61%.

- 17 for stage E, i.e. 15.89%.

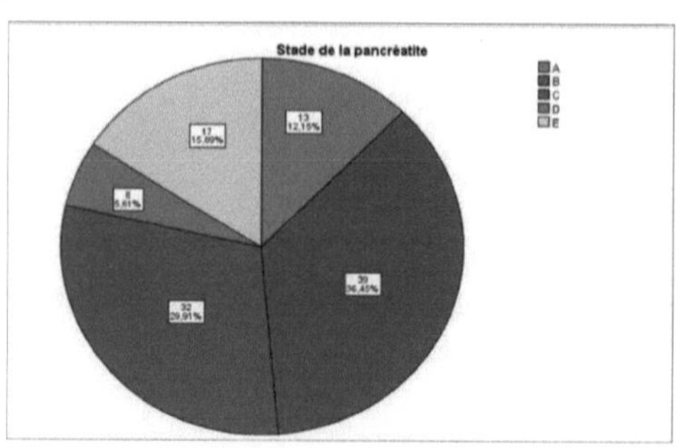

Figure 13: Breakdown by stage of pancreatitis

20

Classifying pancreatitis as oedemato-interstitial and necrotic-haemorrhagic, the rate of necrotising pancreatitis was 21.5% (23 patients).

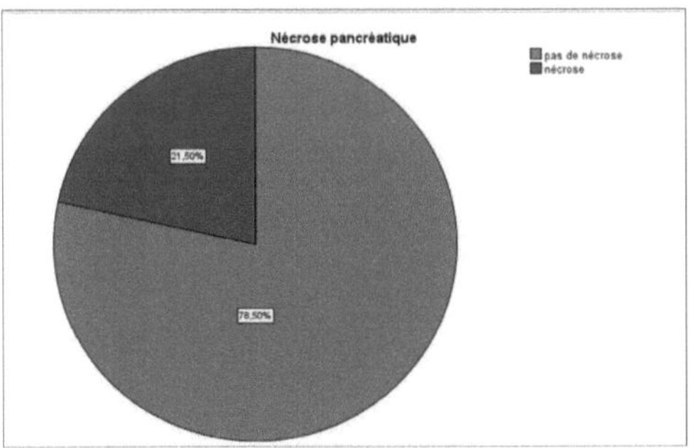

Figure 14: Pancreatic necrosis rate

V. Intraoperative data

1. Appearance of the gall bladder

The intraoperative appearance was consistent with acute cholecystitis in 28 cases (26%).

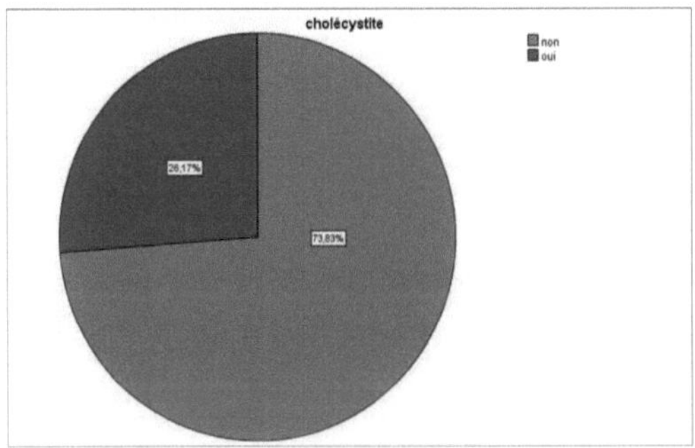

Figure 15: Frequency of acute cholecystitis

2. Dilation of the cystic duct

Intraoperatively, a dilated cystic duct was noted in 14 patients (13%).

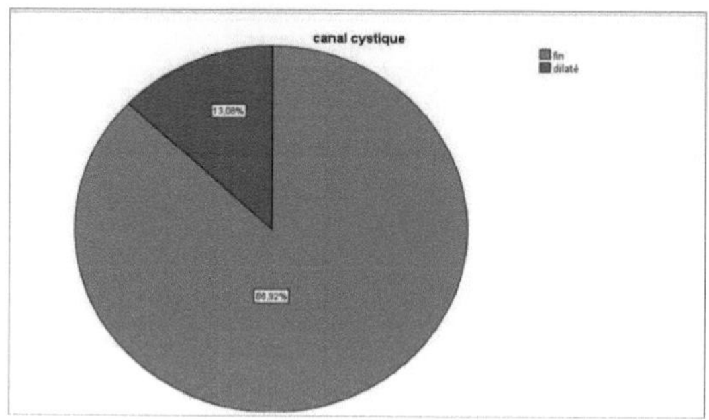

Figure 16: Frequency of cystic duct dilatation

3. CPO data

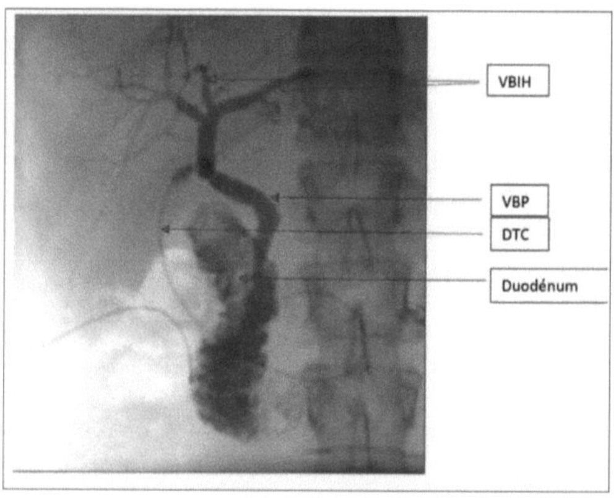

Figure 17: Illustration of a CPO with no anomalies

3.1. Dilatation of the VBP

The diameter of the VBP was approximated by comparing it with the diameter of the trocars. The VBP was dilated in 26.2% (28 patients).

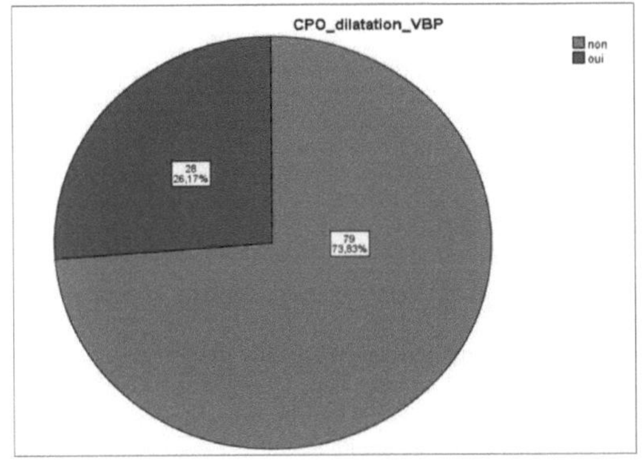

Figure 18: Dilatation rate of the BPV at OPC

3.2. Dilatation of VBIH

Twelve patients (11.2%) had dilated HBV.

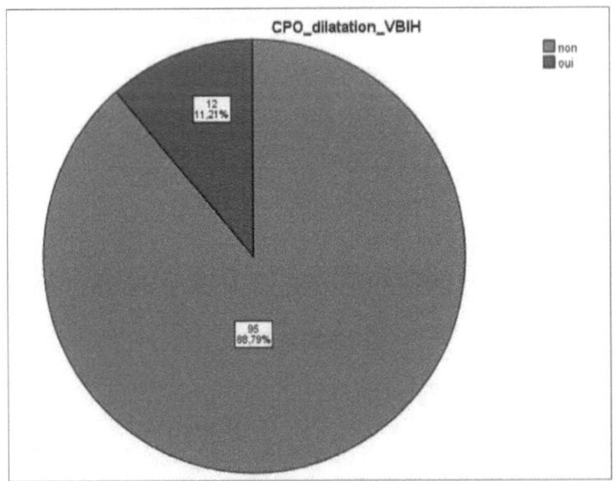

Figure 19: Dilatation rate of HBV at CPO

3.3. Duodenal passage

Duodenal passage was not mentioned in one case. It was early in 72.9% of cases (78 patients), late in 18.7% (20 patients) and absent in 6.5% of OPCs (7).

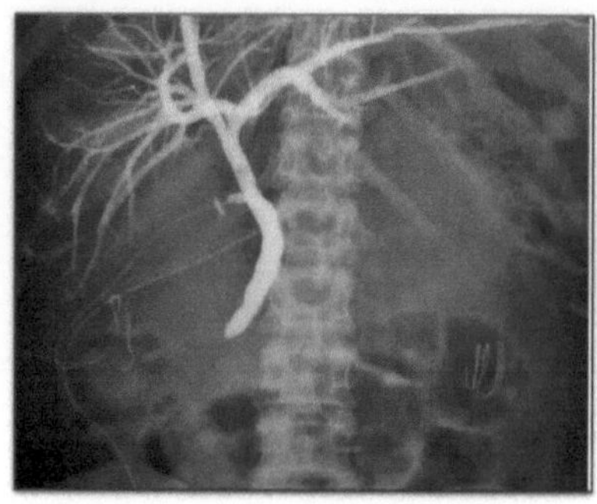

Figure 20: CPO illustrating the absence of duodenal passage

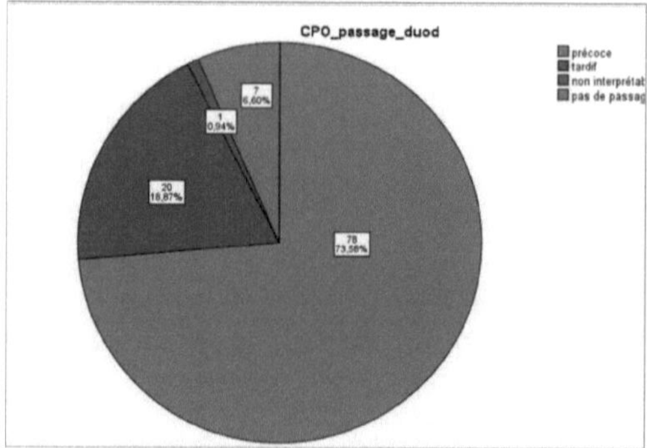

Figure 21: Distribution according to the quality of the duodenal passage

3.4. LVBP

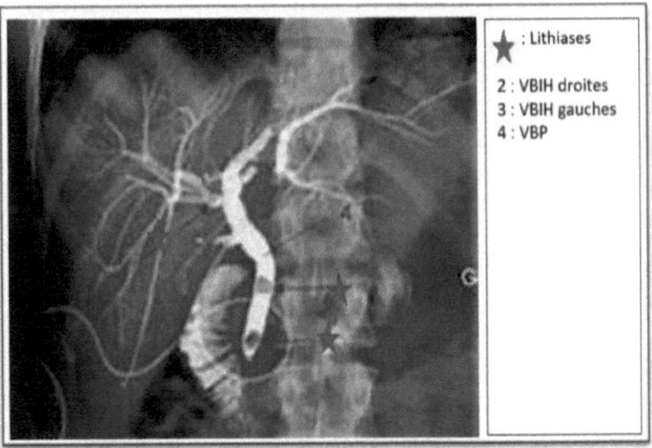

Figure 22: CPO illustrating lacunar images of lithiasis

Eighteen CPOs (16.8%) found a LVBP in the form of a lacunar image.

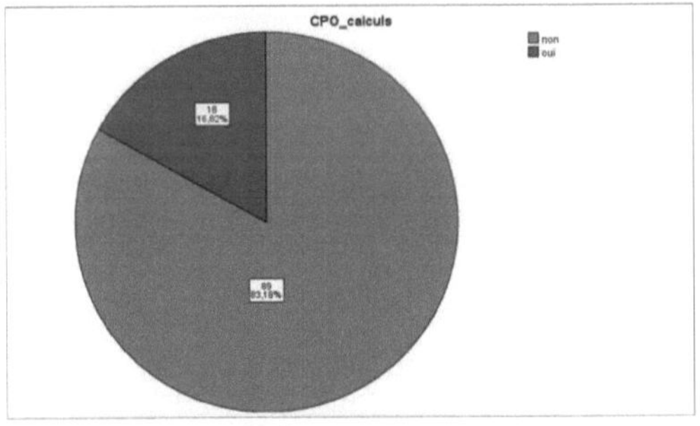

Figure 23: LVBP rate at CPO

4. Gesture

Choleocotomy with stone extraction was performed in 14 patients. The choledochorraphy was semi-ideal in 7 cases and on Kehr drain in the 7 others. The DTC was kept in place in a total of 28 patients. It should be noted that this was the case in one of the following anomalies: dilatation of the VBP, dilatation of the VBIH, poor duodenal passage, difficult interpretation. Postoperative cholangiography was performed in all patients with biliary drainage. In 4 cases, a LVBP was found and an endoscopic sphincterotomy was performed.

B. Analytical study

I. Univariate study

1. Characteristics of the population studied

1.1. Age :

Comparison of the mean age of the two groups showed no significant difference; p = 0.15.

Table 7: Comparison of groups by age

	LVBP Group	Group no LVBP	p
Average	56,71	50,34	0,15
Standard deviation	18,86	17,86	

1.2. Gender :

Three men out of 24 had a LVBP. For women, 18 LVBPs were found in 83 patients. There was no significant difference between the 2 groups (p=0.24).

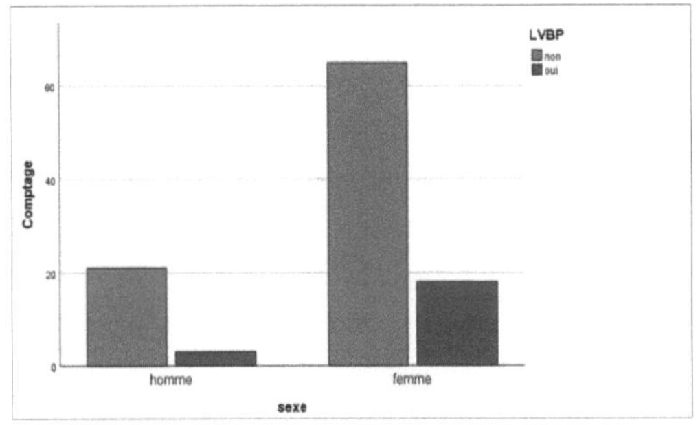

Figure 24: Comparison of groups by gender

1.3. ASA score :

Sixty-seven patients had an ASA score of I, 10 of whom had LVBP. Forty patients had an ASA II score, 11 of whom had a LVBP. There was no statistically significant difference (p=0.17).

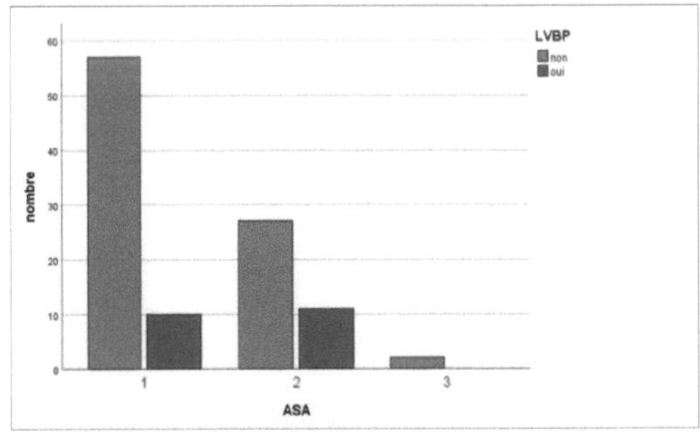

Figure 25: Comparison of groups according to ASA score

1.4. Medical history :

The 2 groups were statistically comparable.

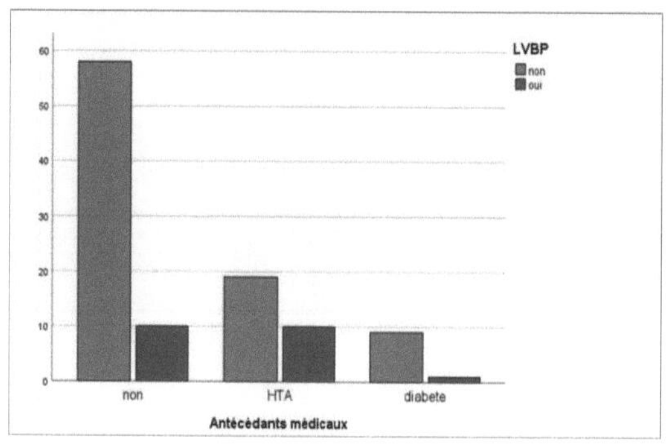

Figure 26: Comparison of groups by medical history

II. Data from the clinical examination

Only one patient had a triad of jaundice, discoloured stools and urine. dark. This patient had LVBP on CPO.Typical liver colic was found in 39 patients (36.4%). LVBP was found in 11 of them and in 10 out of 68 patients without typical liver colic. Statistically, there was no difference between the groups with **p = 0.76**.

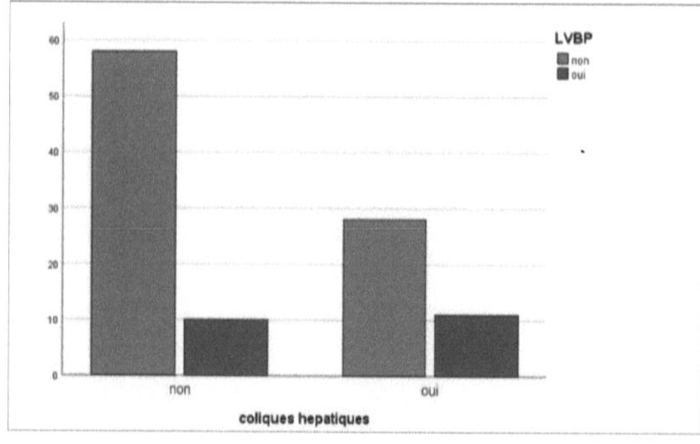

Figure 27: Comparison of groups according to the presence of hepatic colic

Twenty-two patients (20.56%) had severe pancreatitis. LVBP was found in 2 of these patients. The difference between the 2 groups, according to the severity of the pancreatitis, was not statistically significant (**p=0.13**).

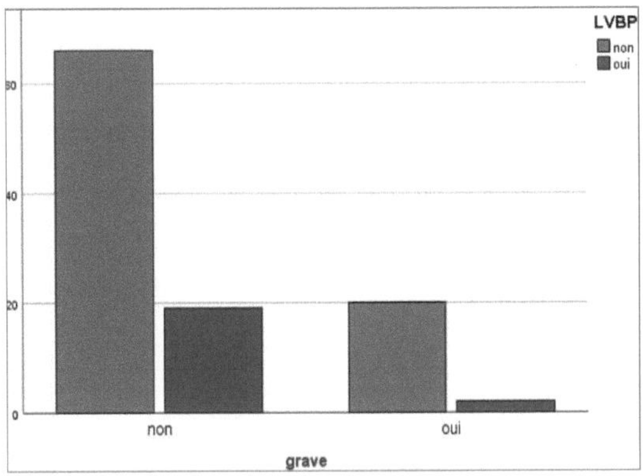

Figure 28: Comparison of groups according to severity of pancreatitis

III.BIOLOGY data

1.Total bilirubin levels

Total bilirubin level was a statistically significant predictor of the presence of LVBP. **P=0,016** By studying the ROC curve, the threshold value of 34.5 mmol/L was selected, with a sensitivity of around 0.6 and a specificity of 0.75.

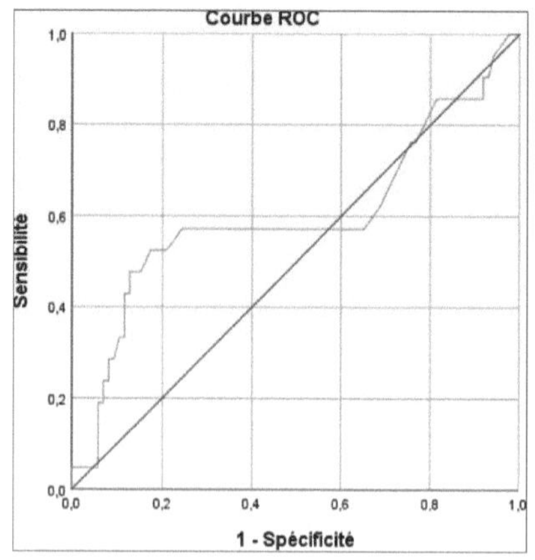

Figure 29: ROC curve analysis for LV

Taking into account this threshold value of total bilirubinemia (TBIL), 65 of the 86 patients without LVBP had a BT level below the TBIL. Twelve of the 21 patients with LVBP had a level above the TSB.

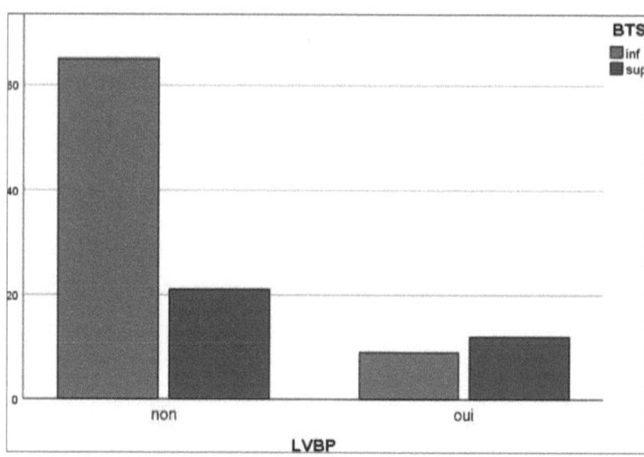

Figure 30: Breakdown of groups by BTS

2. Conjugated bilirubin levels

Conjugated bilirubin level was a statistically significant predictor of LVBP.
P=0,044 By studying the ROC curve, the threshold value of 11.5 mmol/L
was selected, with a sensitivity and specificity of around 0.6.

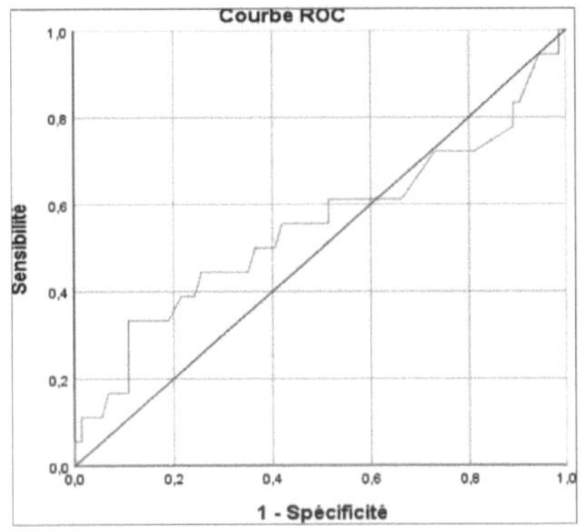

Figure 31: ROC curve analysis for BC

Taking into account this threshold value for conjugated bilirubin (CB), 44
of the 74 patients without LVBP had a CB level below the BCS. Nine of
the 18 patients with LVBP had BC levels above the BCS. In 15 of our
patients, the BC rate was not available.

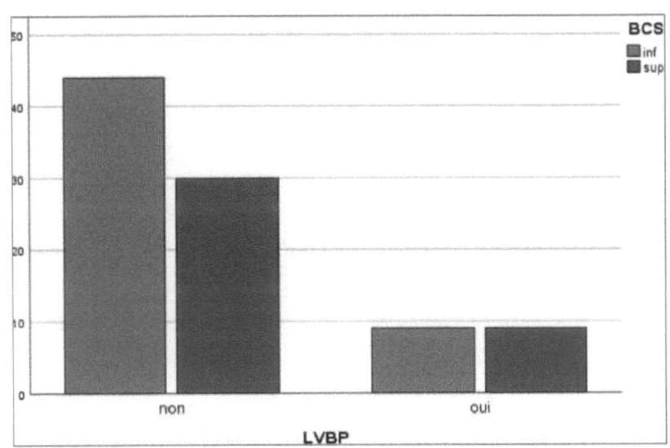

Figure 32: Breakdown of groups by BCS

3.Cytolysis

Cytolysis was not a statistically significant factor in our study. with **p values** of **0.189** and **0.49** respectively for ASAT and ALAT.

4.PAL and GGT

Given their unavailability in the vast majority of cases, their studies could not be reliable.

IV. Imaging data

1. Ultrasound

1.1. Dilatation of the VBP

An LVBP was present at CPO in 13 of the 27 patients with a dilated VBP and in 8 of the 77 without. The difference between the 2 groups was statistically significant with **p=0.00**.

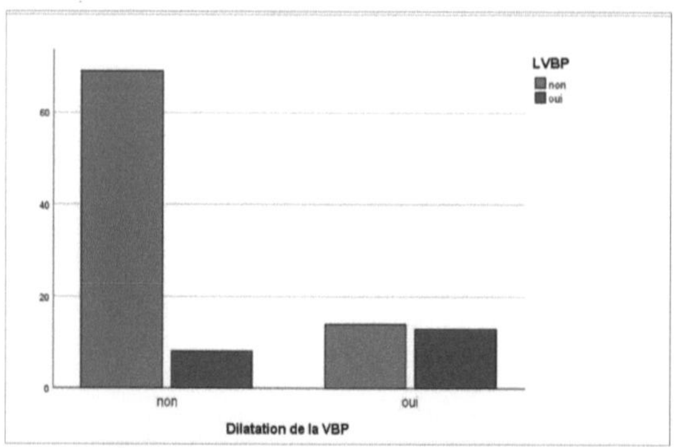

Figure 33: Comparison of groups according to the presence or absence of dilatation of the VBP on ultrasound

1.2. Dilatation of VBIH

Of the 14 cases with dilated HBV, LVBP was present at OPC in 3 and in 18 of the 90 without dilation, with no statistically significant difference **(p=0.57)**.

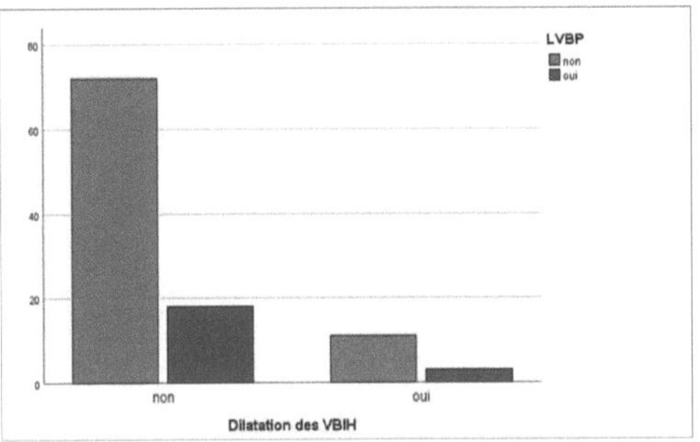

Figure 34: Comparison of groups according to the presence or absence of dilatation of VBIH on ultrasound

2. Computed tomography

2.1. Dilatation of the VBP

LVBP was present at OPC in 11 of the 28 patients with dilated BPV and in 10 of the remaining 79. A significant difference was noted with **p=0.04**.

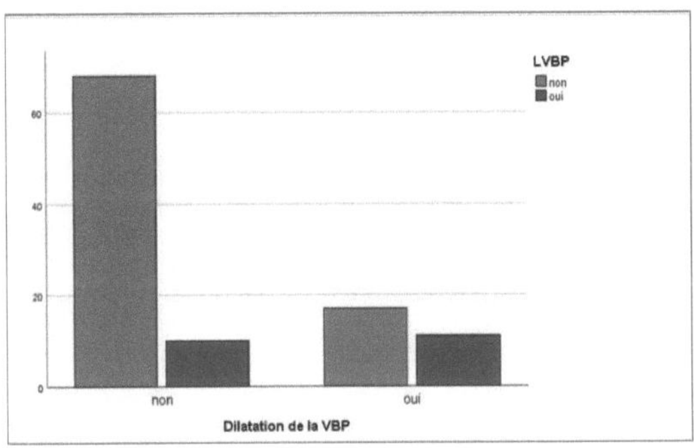

Figure 35: Comparison of groups according to the presence or absence of BPV dilatation on CT scan

2.2. Dilatation of VBIH

Of the 15 cases in which CPO showed dilatation of the HBV, LVBP was present in 3 and in 18 of the remaining 92 with no statistically significant difference (**p=0.60**).

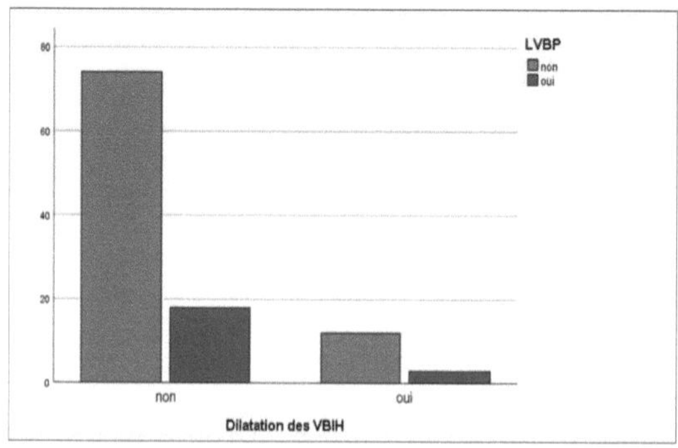

Figure 36: Comparison of groups according to the presence or absence of dilatation of the HBV on CT scan

2.3. Stage of pancreatitis

There was no statistically significant difference between the different stages with regard to the presence or absence of LVBP at CPO.

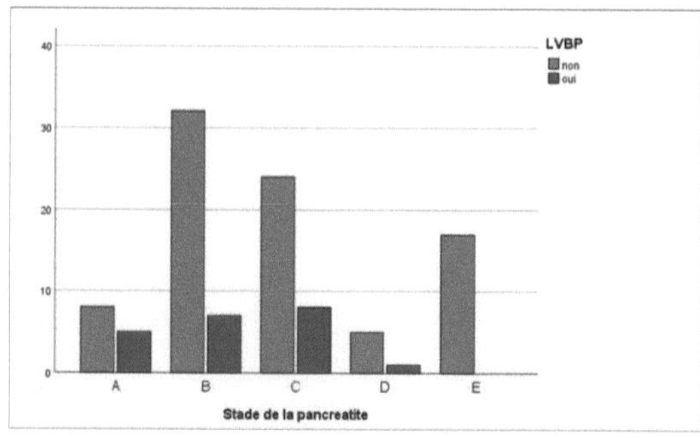

Figure 37: Comparison of groups at different stages of pancreatitis

In the case of necrotic haemorrhagic AP (23 patients), LVBP was detected on CPO in only 1 patient. However, LVBP was found on CPO in 20 out of 80 patients with oedemato-interstitial pancreatitis. The difference was significant at **p=0.028**.

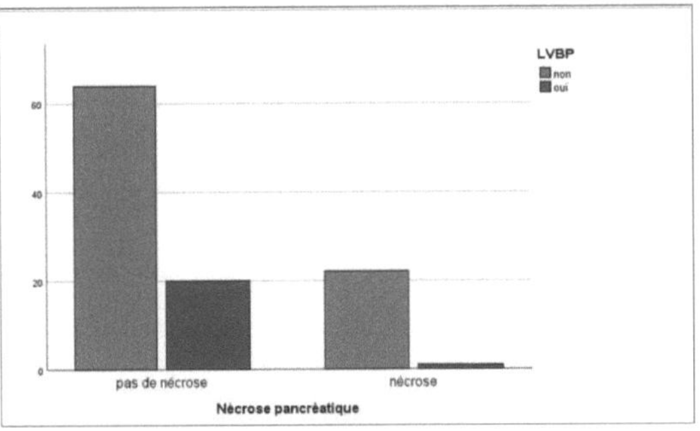

Figure 38: Comparison of groups according to the presence or absence of pancreatic necrosis

V. Intraoperative data

1. Acute cholecystitis

Comparing the 2 groups, there was no significant difference in terms of the presence of LVBP (**p=0.13**).

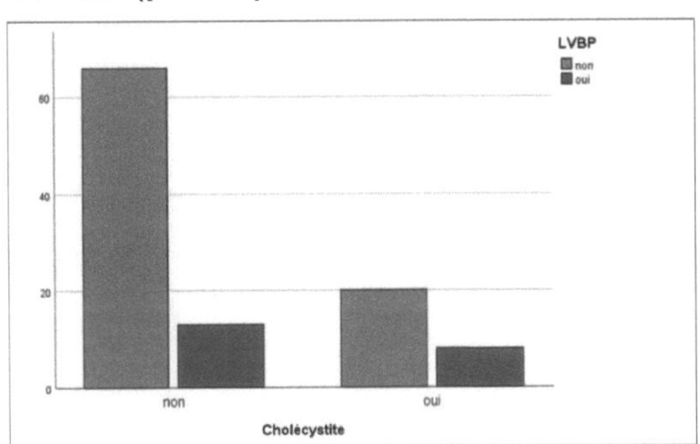

Figure 39: Comparison of groups according to the presence or absence of acute cholecystitis

2.Dilation of the cystic duct

Of the 14 patients in whom we found cystic duct dilatation intraoperatively, 10 had LVBPs compared with 11 of the remaining 82. The difference was statistically significant (**p=0.00**).

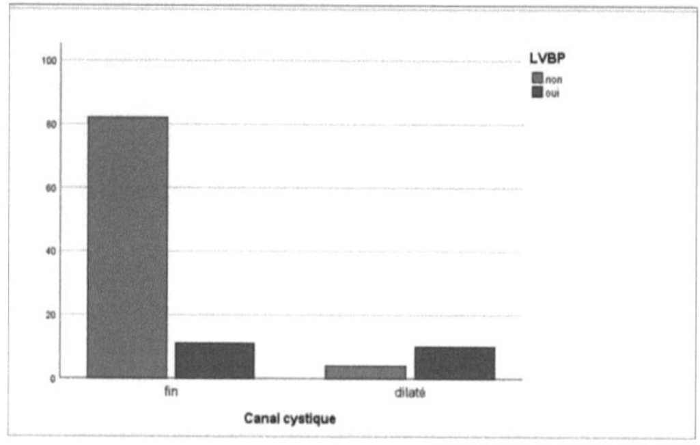

Figure 40: Comparison of groups according to the presence or absence of cystic duct dilatation

C. Multivariate study

Multivariate analysis allowed us to retain only 2 factors: total bilirubin level and dilatation of the VBP on ultrasound. This rate (BT) was set at 34.5 by studying the ROC curve.

D. Score

We established a mathematical translation of the 2 factors (total bilirubin level and dilatation of the VBP on ultrasound) in the form of a simple score in order to test our results.

S = E + 0.03 BT

E = 1 if dilatation of the VBP on ultrasound (more than 6 mm). E = 0 if no dilatation of the VBP on ultrasound.

BT = total bilirubin level in mmol/l

We calculated the score for each case and the results are as follows:

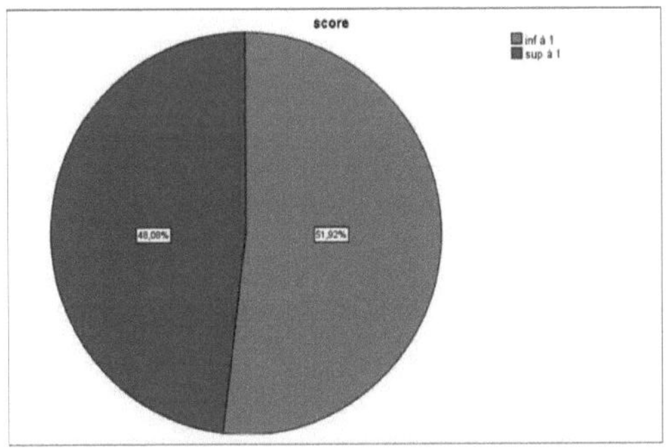

Figure 41: Breakdown by "S" score

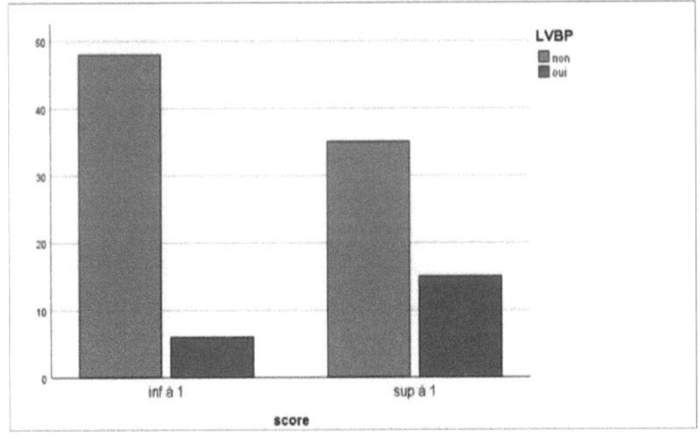

Figure 42: Comparison of groups according to "S" score

Of the 107 cases studied, 6 (05%) had a score of less than 1 with the presence of LVBP on CPO. So, according to our series, more than half of the CPOs could have been avoided (51% had a score of less than 1) with an error rate of around 5%.

DISCUSSION

I. Results

We identified 107 patients with acute pancreatitis of biliary origin who underwent cholecystectomy with OPC. The VBP was found to be empty in 80.4% of cases (86 patients).

The univariate analysis revealed 6 independent factors for the presence of LVBP. These factors are:

• Total bilirubin level.

• Conjugated bilirubin levels.

• Dilatation of the VBP on ultrasound.

• Dilatation of the VBP on CT.

• The stage of the pancreatitis: stages D and E indicate that the VBP is empty.

• Intraoperative dilatation of the cystic duct.

Multivariate analysis allowed us to retain only 2: the total bilirubin level and the dilatation of the VBP on ultrasound. This rate was set at 34.5 by studying the ROC curve.

II. Epidemiology

Three types of gallstone have been described: cholesterol stones, black pigment stones and brown pigment stones. Cholesterol stones account for 80-90% of all gallstones seen in the West (7). Several abnormalities of the liver, gallbladder and intestine are at the root of cholesterol stone formation (10). Bile supersaturated with cholesterol is the main condition leading to stone formation. If other conditions are met, vesicles and microcrystals will appear and macroscopic stones are formed. Stone migration can also temporarily obstruct the sphincter of Oddi and the duct of Wirsung, leading to intra-canal hyperpressure with impaired elimination and reflux of pancreatic secretions. Trypsinogen is thus inadequately activated in the pancreas, causing it to autodigest. The inflammatory response thus initiated leads to the release of cytokines, resulting in direct cytotoxicity and necrosis of the pancreatic gland. Several factors favouring vesicular cholesterol lithiasis have been identified (11). The most frequently cited were age (it is very rare before the age of 20 and its prevalence peaks at around 70), gender (women are twice as likely as men of the same age) and first-degree family history. Between 11,000 and 13,000 new cases are observed in France every year. The incidence is 30/100,000 for men and 20/100,000 for women (4).

III. Predictive factors for LVBP

The International Pancreatology Association and the American Gastroenterology Association recommend that all patients with pancreatitis undergo cholecystectomy as soon as the patient has recovered from symptoms (13,14) The appropriate timing for definitive treatment of patients with non-severe AP has not yet been established, but the current recommendation is to perform cholecystectomy during initial hospitalisation to prevent recurrences and readmissions, which can occur in up to 31% of patients in the first 2 weeks (15,16). Over the past 2 decades, recommendations for preoperative endoscopic assessment and treatment of LVBP have ranged from mandatory endoscopic retrograde cholangiopancreatography (ERCP) in all cases (17) to, more recently, selective preoperative ERCP for stone removal based on clinical presentation and laboratory values. (18,19)

However, the most appropriate method for investigating LVBP and the timing of assessment of the likelihood of bile duct stones in patients with AP has not yet been established. In clinical practice, the decision to perform CPO, MRI, endoscopic ultrasound, laparoscopic ultrasound or endoscopic retrograde cholangiopancreatography (ERCP) is often based on biological and radiological criteria; and depends on the resources and availability of diagnostic methods at the medical centre.

To improve the approach in patients at risk of LVBP, the predictors proposed by ASGE have been extensively studied: among them VBP >6mm with a sensitivity of 64.7% to 90% and specificity of 23% to 76.1%, total bilirubin between 1.8 and 4mg /dL, with a sensitivity of 19% to 61% and specificity of 44% to 85%. (20). In our study, these 2 factors were predictive of the presence of LVBP and in particular a total bilirubin level greater than 34.5 mmol/L (i.e. 2mg/dL).

The prevalence of PVLB increases with age (21). A previous study showed that among patients referred for endoscopic ultrasound for assessment of LV stones, the prevalence increased to 32% in patients over 70 years of age compared with 14% in patients under 70 years of age (22). In our series, the most common age group was between 33 and 69 years (58.9%). Another study showed that a VBP width greater than 6 mm had a significant positive correlation with LVBP (23).

In addition, GGT levels have been shown to be an important predictor of LVBP (24,25). A study by Chan et al. confirmed that an elevated serum total bilirubin level on day two is predictive of persistent PBV stones in patients with biliary pancreatitis(26).

Table 8: LV rate on the second day of hospitalisation as a predictor of LVBP according to Chan et al (26)

TABLE 2. *Predictive Value of Serum Total Bilirubin on Hospital Day 2*

	Total Bilirubin ≥ 5 mg/dL	Total Bilirubin ≥ 4 mg/dL	Total Bilirubin ≥ 3 mg/dL	Total Bilirubin ≥ 2 mg/dL
Sensitivity	33%	39%	44%	50%
Specificity	97%	95%	93%	85%
Positive predictive value	55%	44%	40%	27%
Negative predictive value	93%	93%	94%	94%
P value	0.0004	<0.0001	<0.0001	<0.0001

By integrating the patient's age in years, the GGT value in U/L and the diameter > 6 mm of VBP on ultrasound, Khoury et al. were able to generate a score of simple diagnosis. This method can provide practitioners with a simple bedside tool to classify patients into different groups and offer them the appropriate treatment while avoiding unnecessary investigations. For example, for Khoury, a score ranging from 9 to 41 has a high sensitivity (82% to 100%) of no LVBP, suggesting that this group may not benefit from expensive and invasive investigative procedures and can be managed conservatively without endoscopic intervention (27). In our study, the two predictive factors for persistence of LVBP after pancreatitis were increased total bilirubin levels and dilatation of more than 6 mm of the VBP on abdominal ultrasound. The surgical treatment of acute biliary pancreatitis has also evolved, particularly in the era of minimally invasive techniques. Studies have shown that with the increasing use of laparoscopic techniques, combined with preoperative or postoperative ERCP, hospital stays and investigations of the BPV have decreased considerably in recent years. (28)

IV. Intraoperative cholangiography

1. Interest

Because of the perceived risk of stone retention, the traditional teaching has been that patients who do not meet the criteria for preoperative ERCP should undergo mandatory intraoperative cholangiography at the time of surgical gallbladder removal. (28,29)

CPO has a sensitivity of 76% to 100% and a specificity of 96% to 100% in the diagnosis of LVBP (30). Although MRI and CPO have similar sensitivity and specificity, CPO has the advantage that it can only be performed during cholecystectomy, which may reduce waiting days for the surgery and hospital stay by eliminating the time interval between the VBP study (MRI) and surgery.Intraoperative cholangiography is generally recommended during cholecystectomy to detect any stones (31).

False positive results due to air bubbles are inevitable and can affect up to 35% of patients (32). However, we were increasingly impressed by the rarity with which routine CPO detected stones at the time of surgery in patients with acute biliary pancreatitis.

2. Disadvantages

In more than three quarters of patients with biliary AP, the stone is not found in the PVB, which is explained by the fact that the majority of stones are small, less than 5 mm in size, thus facilitating spontaneous passage. (27,33) Our study shows similar results. Of the 107 CPOs, 86 showed no LVBP (80.4%). On the other hand, CPO results in a longer operating time (89 vs. 68 minutes for laparoscopy [P 0.0001]) and a longer postoperative hospital stay (3.8 vs. 2.0 days [P 0.007]), without any effect on the incidence of residual calculi. (34)

Sajid et al analysed three randomised controlled trials evaluating the effect of CPO on operating time and concluded that CPO results in longer operating times (35). For this reason, in our practice, we have become extremely selective in the performance of CPO in patients with acute biliary pancreatitis to the point where it is now performed very rarely. The aim of this study was to document the outcomes of a management regimen in patients with acute biliary pancreatitis that does not include CPO.

5. Other resources

5.1 Ultrasound

Abdominal ultrasound can be used to look for vesicular lithiasis and signs of lithiasis of the main bile duct. It can detect vesicular calculi with a sensitivity of 90%, but this falls considerably in the diagnosis of choledocholithic calculi (sensitivity between 50 and 80%) (36).

2. Computed tomography

Computed tomography detects vesicular lithiasis less easily, with a sensitivity of 60-87% (36).

3. Magnetic resonance imaging

Magnetic resonance cholangio-pancreatography (MRCP) is a reliable means of diagnosing lithiasis of the main bile duct, with a specificity of 94% (37).

4. Endoscopic ultrasound

Endoscopic ultrasound and MRCP have the same specificity (94%) for diagnosing LVBP. However, endoscopic ultrasound is better at identifying small stones (< 6 mm), with a sensitivity of 90%. This sensitivity is 82% for MRCP (36), and endoscopic retrograde cholangio-pancreatography (ERCP). The advantage of the latter is that it also allows sphincterotomy. endoscopy at the same time.

CONCLUSION

In 30-70% of cases, AP is caused by lithiasis. All patients with biliary pancreatitis should have a cholecystectomy as soon as the patient has recovered from symptoms, to prevent recurrence. The most appropriate method for studying LVBP and the timing of the assessment of the likelihood of common bile duct stones in patients with AP has not yet been established. Magnetic resonance cholangiopancreatography is the most widely used imaging technique, but in our country, given the difficulty of its availability, intraoperative cholangiography is still the most commonly used method for detecting any LVBP. In more than three quarters of patients with biliary AP, the stone is not present. not found in the VBP.In our practice, we have become extremely selective in the performance of CPO in patients with acute biliary pancreatitis. To improve the approach in patients at risk of LVBP, predictors have been proposed by the ASGE and have been extensively studied by several teams. The aim of this study was to review the formal indication for CPO in this condition by investigating factors predictive of the presence of LVBP following acute pancreatitis of lithiasis origin. We studied the files of 107 patients who met the previously established criteria. The univariate analysis revealed 6 independent factors for the presence of LVBP These include: total bilirubin level, conjugated bilirubin level, dilatation of the PVB on ultrasound, dilatation of the PVB on CT scan, stage of pancreatitis (stages D and E being in favour of a vacant PVB) and intraoperative dilatation of the cystic duct. Multivariate analysis allowed us to retain only 2: the total bilirubin level and the dilatation of the VBP on ultrasound. This rate was set at 34.5 by studying the ROC curve.We have established a mathematical translation of these 2 factors in the form of a simple score to test our results.

S = E + 0.03 BT

$E = 1$ if dilatation of the VBP on ultrasound (more than 6 mm). $E = 0$ if no dilatation of the VBP on ultrasound.
BT = total bilirubin level in mmol/l.
A score greater than or equal to 1 would indicate that intraoperative cholangiography should be performed during cholecystectomy.

So, according to our series, **more than half of all CPOs could have been avoided. with an error rate of around 5%.**

The limitations of our study were the sample size and the missing biological markers of cholestasis, namely GGT and LAP, which are frequently found in the literature. This prompts us to carry out similar trials, multicentre and prospective studies, in order to standardise the management of patients presenting with a The aim is to reduce the number of cases of acute biliary pancreatitis caused by lithiasis in our country, and to limit as far as possible the use of CPO, which is still over-used and not without risks. We therefore call for prospective studies using a suitable methodology to verify, and even improve, this score.

REFERENCES

1. Aussilhou B, Dokmak S, Sauvanet A. Acute pancreatitis. J Eur Urgences Réanimation. March 2013;25(1):32-40.

2. Shen HN, Wang WC, Lu CL, Li CY. Effects of Gender on Severity, Management and Outcome in Acute Biliary Pancreatitis. Einwaechter H, editor. PLoS ONE. 28 Feb 2013;8(2):e57504.

3. Lévy P, Boruchowicz A, Hastier P, Pariente A, Thévenot T, Frossard JL, et al. Diagnostic criteria in predicting a biliary origin of acute pancreatitis in the era of endoscopic ultrasound: Multicentre prospective evaluation of 213 patients. Pancreatology. Jan 2005;5(4-5):450-6.

4. Bougard M, Barbier L, Godart B, Le Bayon-Bréard AG, Marques F, Salamé E. Management of acute lithiasis pancreatitis. J Chir Visceral. Apr 2019;156(2):130-42.

5. Buxbaum JL, Abbas Fehmi SM, Sultan S, Fishman DS, Qumseya BJ, Cortessis VK, et al. ASGE guideline on the role of endoscopy in the evaluation and management of choledocholithiasis. Gastrointest Endosc. June 2019;89(6):1075-1105.e15.

6. Maple JT, Ben-Menachem T, Anderson MA, Appalaneni V, Banerjee S, Cash BD, et al. The role of endoscopy in the evaluation of suspected choledocholithiasis. Gastrointest Endosc. Jan 2010;71(1):1-9.

7. Payen JL, Muscari F, Vibert É, Ernst O, Pelletier G. Biliary lithiasis. Presse Médicale. June 2011;40(6):567-80.

8. Varghese JC, Liddell RP, Farrell MA, Murray FE, Osborne DH, Lee MJ. Diagnostic Accuracy of Magnetic Resonance Cholangiopancreatography and Ultrasound Compared with Direct Cholangiography in the Detection of Choledocholithiasis. Clin Radiol. Jan

2000;55(1):25-35.

9. Catheline JM, Borie F, Champault G, Millat B. Catheline JM, Borie F, Champault G, Millat B. Intraoperative diagnosis of lithiasis of the main bile duct. Monographie de l'Association Francaise de Chirurgie sur la lithiase de la voie biliaire principale 1999;37-50. In.

10. Portincasa P, Moschetta A, Palasciano G. Cholesterol gallstone disease. The Lancet. July 2006;368(9531):230-9.

11. Lambou-Gianoukos S, Heller SJ. Lithogenesis and Bile Metabolism. Surg Clin North Am. Dec 2008;88(6):1175-94.

12. Roberts SE, Akbari A, Thorne K, Atkinson M, Evans PA. The incidence of acute pancreatitis: impact of social deprivation, alcohol consumption, seasonal and demographic factors. Aliment Pharmacol Ther. Sep 2013;38(5):539-48.

13. Uhl W, Warshaw A, Imrie C, Bassi C, McKay CJ, Lankisch PG, et al. IAP Guidelines for the surgical management of acute pancreatitis. Pancreatology. 1 Jan 2002;2(6):565-73.

14. Tenner S, Baillie J, DeWitt J, Vege SS. American College of Gastroenterology Guideline: Management of Acute Pancreatitis. Am J Gastroenterol. Sep 2013;108(9):1400-15.

15. Park JG, Kim KB, Han JH, Yoon SM, Chae HB, Youn SJ, et al. The Usefulness of Early Endoscopic Ultrasonography in Acute Biliary Pancreatitis with Undetectable Choledocholithiasis on Multidetector Computed Tomography. Korean J Gastroenterol. 4 Oct 2016;68(4):202-9.

16. Anderloni A, Repici A. Role and timing of endoscopy in acute biliary pancreatitis. World J Gastroenterol WJG. 28 Oct 2015;21(40):11205-8.

17. Fan ST, Lai E, Mok F, Lo CM, Zheng SS, Wong J. Early Treatment of Acute Biliary Pancreatitis by Endoscopic Papillotomy. N Engl J Med. 28

Jan 1993;328(4):228-32.

18. Fölsch UR, Nitsche R, Lüdtke R, Hilgers RA, Creutzfeldt W. Early ERCP and Papillotomy Compared with Conservative Treatment for Acute Biliary Pancreatitis. N Engl J Med. 23 Jan 1997;336(4):237-42.

19. Soetikno RM, Carr-Locke DL. Endoscopic management of acute gallstone pancreatitis. Gastrointest Endosc Clin N Am. Jan 1998;8(1):1-12.

20. He H, Tan C, Wu J, Dai N, Hu W, Zhang Y, et al. Accuracy of ASGE high-risk criteria in evaluation of patients with suspected common bile duct stones. Gastrointest Endosc. Sep 2017;86(3):525-32.

21. Barkun AN, Barkun JS, Fried GM, Ghitulescu G, Steinmetz O, Pham C, et al. Useful Predictors of Bile Duct Stones in Patients Undergoing Laparoscopic Cholecystectomy: Ann Surg. July 1994;220(1):32-9.

22. Prat F, Meduri B, Ducot B, Chiche R, Salimbeni-Bartolini R, Pelletier G. Prediction of Common Bile Duct Stones by Noninvasive Tests: Ann Surg. March 1999;229(3):362-8.

23. Nárvaez Rivera RM, González González JA, Monreal Robles R, García Compean D, Paz Delgadillo J, Garza Galindo AA, et al. Accuracy of ASGE criteria for the prediction of choledocholithiasis. Rev Esp Enfermedades Dig [Internet]. 2016 [cited 29 August 2022];108. Available at: https://online.reed.es/fichaArticulo.aspx?iarf=683764745239-413275192166

24. Yang MH, Chen TH, Wang SE, Tsai YF, Su CH, Wu CW, et al. Biochemical predictors for absence of common bile duct stones in patients undergoing laparoscopic cholecystectomy. Surg Endosc. Jul 2008;22(7):1620-4.

25. Peng WK, Sheikh Z, Paterson-Brown S, Nixon SJ. Role of liver

function tests in predicting common bile duct stones in acute calculous cholecystitis. Br J Surg. 20 Sep 2005;92(10):1241-7.

26. Chan T, Yaghoubian A, Rosing D, Lee E, Lewis RJ, Stabile BE, et al. Total Bilirubin is a Useful Predictor of Persisting Common Bile Duct Stone in Gallstone Pancreatitis. Am Surg. Oct 2008;74(10):977-80.

27. Khoury T, Kadah A, Mahamid M, Mari A, Sbeit W. Bedside score predicting retained common bile duct stone in acute biliary pancreatitis. World J Clin Cases. 26 Apr 2020;8(8):1414-23.

28. Schwesinger WH, Page CP, Gross GWW, Miller JE, Strodel WE, Sirinek KR. Biliary Pancreatitis: The Era of Laparoscopic Cholecystectomy. Arch Surg [Internet].1Oct 1998[cited 15 Aug 2022];133(10). Available at: http://archsurg.jamanetwork.com/article.aspx?doi=10.1001/archs urg.133.10.1103

29. Chang L, Lo SK, Stabile BE, Lewis RJ, de Virgilio C. Gallstone Pancreatitis: A Prospective Study on the Incidence of Cholangitis and Clinical Predictors of Retained Common Bile Duct Stones. Am J Gastroenterol. Apr 1998;93(4):527-31.

30. Gurusamy KS, Giljaca V, Takwoingi Y, Higgie D, Poropat G, Štimac D, et al. Endoscopic retrograde cholangiopancreatography versus intraoperative cholangiography for diagnosis of common bile duct stones. Cochrane Hepato- Biliary Group, editor. Cochrane Database Syst Rev [Internet]. 26 Feb 2015 [cited 29 Aug 2022]; Available from: https://doi.wiley.com/10.1002/14651858.CD010339.pub2

31. Telem DA, Bowman K, Hwang J, Chin EH, Nguyen SQ, Divino CM. Selective Management of Patients with Acute Biliary Pancreatitis. J Gastrointest Surg. Dec 2009;13(12):2183-8.

32. Varadarajulu S, Eloubeidi MA, Wilcox CM, Hawes RH, Cotton PB. Do all patients with abnormal intraoperative cholangiogram merit endoscopic retrograde cholangiopancreatography? Surg Endosc. May 2006;20(5):801-5.

33. Tranter S, Thompson M. Spontaneous passage of bile duct stones: frequency of occurrence and relation to clinical presentation. Ann R Coll Surg Engl :4.

34. Bennion R. Effect of Intraoperative Cholangiography During Cholecystectomy on Outcome After Gallstone Pancreatitis. J Gastrointest Surg. August 2002;6(4):575-81.

35. Sajid M, Leaver C, Haider Z, Worthington T, Karanjia N, Singh K. Routine on-table cholangiography during cholecystectomy: a systematic review. Ann R Coll Surg Engl. Sep 1, 2012;94(6):375-80.

36. Șurlin V. Imaging tests for accurate diagnosis of acute biliary pancreatitis. World J Gastroenterol. 2014;20(44):16544.

37. IAP/APA evidence-based guidelines for the management of acute pancreatitis. Pancreatology. july 2013;13(4):e1-15.

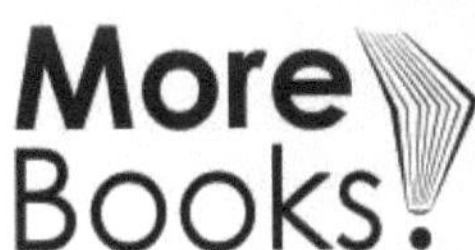

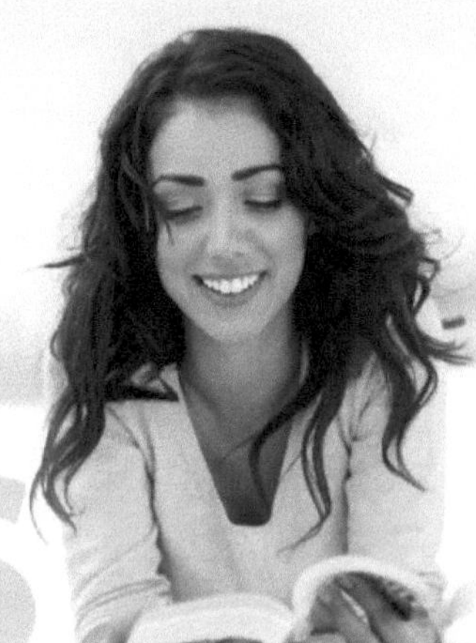

yes
I want morebooks!

Buy your books fast and straightforward online - at one of world's fastest growing online book stores! Environmentally sound due to Print-on-Demand technologies.

Buy your books online at
www.morebooks.shop

Kaufen Sie Ihre Bücher schnell und unkompliziert online – auf einer der am schnellsten wachsenden Buchhandelsplattformen weltweit! Dank Print-On-Demand umwelt- und ressourcenschonend produziert.

Bücher schneller online kaufen
www.morebooks.shop

info@omniscriptum.com
www.omniscriptum.com

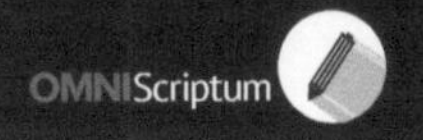

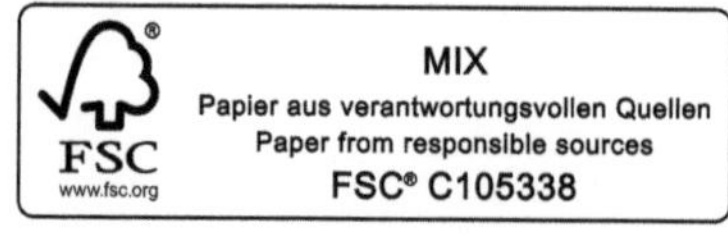

Printed by Books on Demand GmbH, Norderstedt / Germany